C25K

The Couch to 5K Beginner Running Program

Matthew C. Lee

Contents

The Purpose of the Book

Couch to 5K is a pretty straightforward running program and you *can* do it without a book – after all I did it without a book and so have countless others. But the program's simplicity leaves a lot of questions to be answered. After completing the program I've had a lot of questions about it from people who were either doing the program or considering it. This book is an attempt to answer some of these common questions. This will make starting the program easier and – just as importantly – it will make finishing the program easier! I suggest that you read this book once through before you begin the program. This will give you an overview of Couch to 5K and how it works. Then keep the book on hand to answer questions that you may have as you progress through the program.

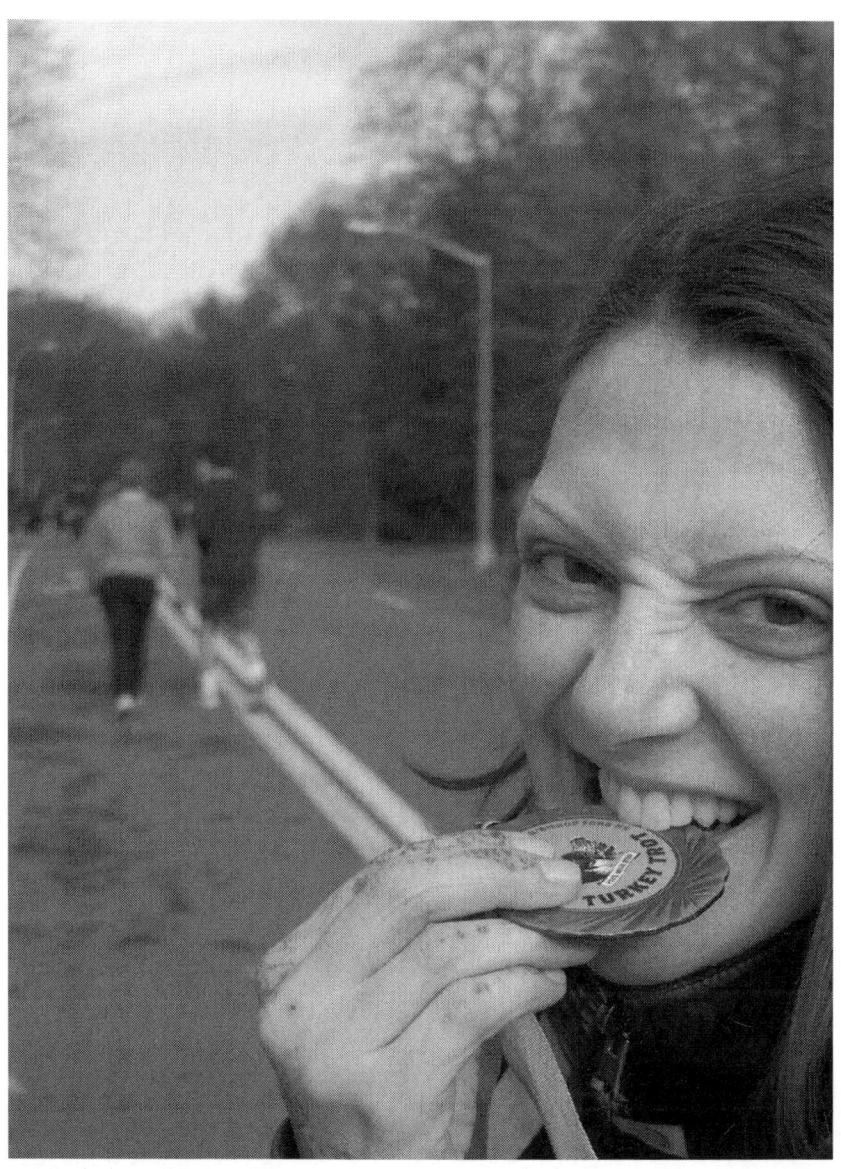

Couch to 5K will help you reach the finish. (Pixonomy – CC BY-ND 2.0)

My Story

Growing up I was an active, even athletic kid. I played soccer, hockey, basketball and rugby at various points throughout elementary, middle and high school. I was always a naturally good runner but I never really trained or competed as a runner – apart from middle school track and cross country. But I was always running as part of the conditioning for the other sports I played. I was in better-than-average shape and I was faster than most kids.

Fast forward to university and everything changed for me. I became focussed on my school work and stopped playing sports. Also, after growing up eating healthy, I started eating pretty terribly when presented with fried foods and ice cream at the university meal hall. I quickly put on weight and got out of shape. It would be almost 10 years before I became active again. That's not to say that I didn't try to get active sooner. A handful of times I decided I was going to get in shape. I even started running a few times, but it never lasted more than a few weeks.

At age 28 I was obese. I didn't feel obese though. In my mind I was still that 18-year-old athlete. Then I went to try on my suit before a wedding – a suit that I bought when I had reached the point that I thought would be my largest – and I found it wouldn't fit. It wasn't an earth shattering realization, but it provided me with a wake-up call and I decided that things needed to change.

I started to eat better and began watching my calories – the pounds started to slip away. But I didn't just want to lose weight; I wanted to get in shape. I started doing an at-home workout program and had good results. This was a start, but I wanted a goal to work towards. I decided that I wanted to run a 5K race. I had heard about the Couch to 5K program before but I had always ignored it and tried to do harder programs (after all I still thought I was an athlete). But this time I decided to give it a try.

I can't tell you how happy I am with that decision. A short while into the program I was already able to do a short run, completing a 3k race. By week nine I was ready for the real deal and I completed a 5K race. I'm no longer overweight and I run regularly, sometimes covering 300 Km or more in a month – the equivalent of more than 60 5K runs. A few months after completing Couch to 5K I completed a half marathon and I completed a marathon soon after. In between these events I ran more races than I can remember off the top of my head. There's really no limit to what I might do with the ability that the Couch to 5K program has given me.

A Brief History of C25K

In his early twenties Josh Clark tried to take up running, but even as a self-described "reasonably fit" guy he found the experience painful. In spite of this he pushed himself through the pain and after a few weeks it became something enjoyable. According to Clark, running became pleasant and even meditative for him. Clark wrote about the experience, saying "it became something that I looked forward to, that gave me energy and, as a happy byproduct, also happened to keep me fit and healthy."

As a newly converted runner Clark became an evangelist for the sport, encouraging others to take it up. But he realized that not everyone would be prepared to simply push through the pain. So Clarke developed a gradual program to ease people into running. The Couch to 5K program was designed with Clark's mother in mind. At the time she was 50 and didn't exercise because she hated it, but she wanted to improve her health. The program was a success for her. As Clark said, "I couldn't have been more pleased when the program worked for her."

Enthusiastic to help others become runners, Clark set up his own website for new runners in the early days of widespread Internet availability. The Couch to 5K program was the focus of this website. In 1996 the Couch to 5K program was featured on the website

Cool Running. Cool Running has gone on to become the longest-running commercial website devoted to running and the site continues to feature Couch to 5K prominently. Cool Running has even developed a Couch to 5K app and other running programs to complement it.

Since 1996 countless people have become runners with the help of the Couch to 5K program. You can find podcasts, fan sites and translations of the program into at least 28 languages including Arabic, Chinese and Swahili. And the reason that Couch to 5K is so popular is simple: it works!

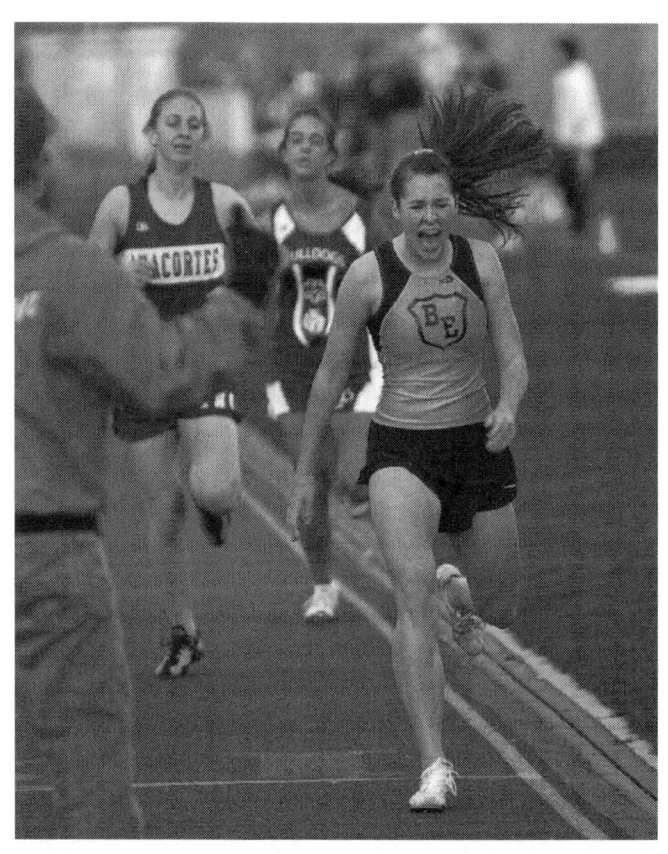

Couch to 5K is about pushing your body, without hurting your body.
(Philo Norlund – CC BY 2.0)

The Philosophy of C25K

According to Josh Clark, the Couch to 5K program was designed according to five basic principles: eliminate pain, welcome newcomers, deliver early victories, make it easy and rewarding, and not everyone wants to be a power user.

Eliminate Pain

No pain, no gain is a common cliché in the fitness world. Advocates of this philosophy believe that you need to push yourself to your limits if you want to see results. But the Couch to 5K philosophy is gain without the pain. The idea is that running shouldn't be too hard or else you'll quit. That's exactly what my experience was in the past. I tried taking up running a handful of times over the years but I could never stick with it. The reason? I was pushing myself too hard, too early. I forgot that I was out of shape and would jump into an intense program without proper preparation. I'd end up quitting either because I found it miserable or because I'd push myself to the point of injury. With Couch to 5K you will push your limits without exceeding them, so you'll see improvements without the pain.

Welcome Newcomers

Most of the people I've met who have completed the Couch to 5K program had never run before. In fact many had no athletic background at all. Personally, I hadn't run competitively since middle school. The Couch to 5K program is simple and straightforward. It avoids runners' jargon and technicalities, sticking to the bare basics of running. You don't need to have run before to do the program, in fact you really don't need to know anything about running before you start it.

Deliver Early Victories

My first week of Couch to 5K was one of my most rewarding weeks. In that week I didn't run for any longer than 60 seconds at a time, but the feeling of accomplishment was on par with completing my first 5K. The goals of the program are reasonable so you will have the satisfaction of accomplishing something early on. This provides motivation and will give you a reason to keep going.

Make It Easy and Rewarding

As Josh Clark said about the Couch to 5K program, "we are creatures of inertia; we need carrots to get moving." The victories come early in the program, but they keep coming as well. Each week will give you a new challenge that you can reasonably expect to accomplish.

Not Everyone Wants to Be a Power User

Not everyone who completes the Couch to 5K program will become a competitive runner or move on to longer distances. Some will be content to just go for a morning jog on a regular basis. But others will want to move on to greater challenges. Whether you just want to be able to run for 30 minutes or you want to run a marathon, the Couch to 5K program will prepare you for either path. So if you just want to be a casual runner you don't need to worry about being overwhelmed, but at the same time you can rest assured that the program will give you a solid foundation if you want to push yourself further.

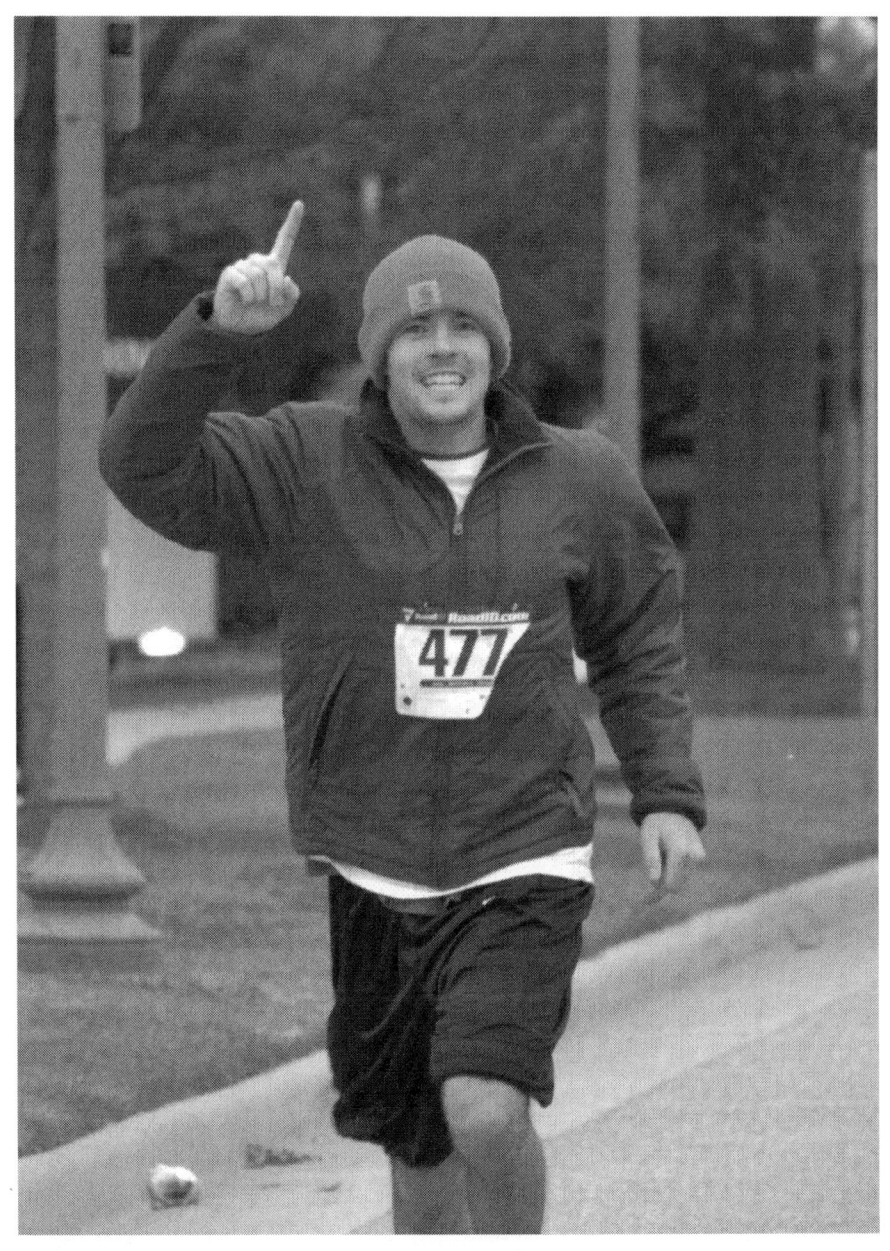

Above all else, running's about having fun. (Tony Alter – CC BY 2.0)

Before You Start

The Couch to 5K program is challenging, but it will ease you into running. For most people there won't be any health concerns associated with the program, but only a physician can tell you this definitively. Talk to your physician to see if the program is right for you. If you have certain medical conditions your doctor may advise against pursuing the program immediately. Even if you think you're in decent shape it's worth getting a checkup. Most of us who have neglected our fitness routines have also neglected our regular visits to the doctor so you may be overdue anyway.

Once a doctor gives you the okay to start the program you're ready to get down to business. If you're really serious about the program (and you should be!) I recommend registering for a 5K race that's scheduled to take place not long after you expect to finish the program. This will give you a clear goal to work toward. If you want even more motivation find a friend, family member, boyfriend, girlfriend, spouse, etc. who wants to run the 5K with you. If you train together you can keep each other accountable. If you can't rope anyone into your plans look to the internet for help – there's no shortage of forums and social networks connecting runners with common goals. Internal motivation can also be a big motivator to get you through the program. Before you start the program, think about why you want to do it. Maybe you just want to be in better shape, maybe you want to improve your health or you just like the challenge of competing in a 5K race. Whatever your reasons, write them down so you remember them when the going gets tough. Post them on your mirror, your desk, the fridge or somewhere else where you'll see them regularly.

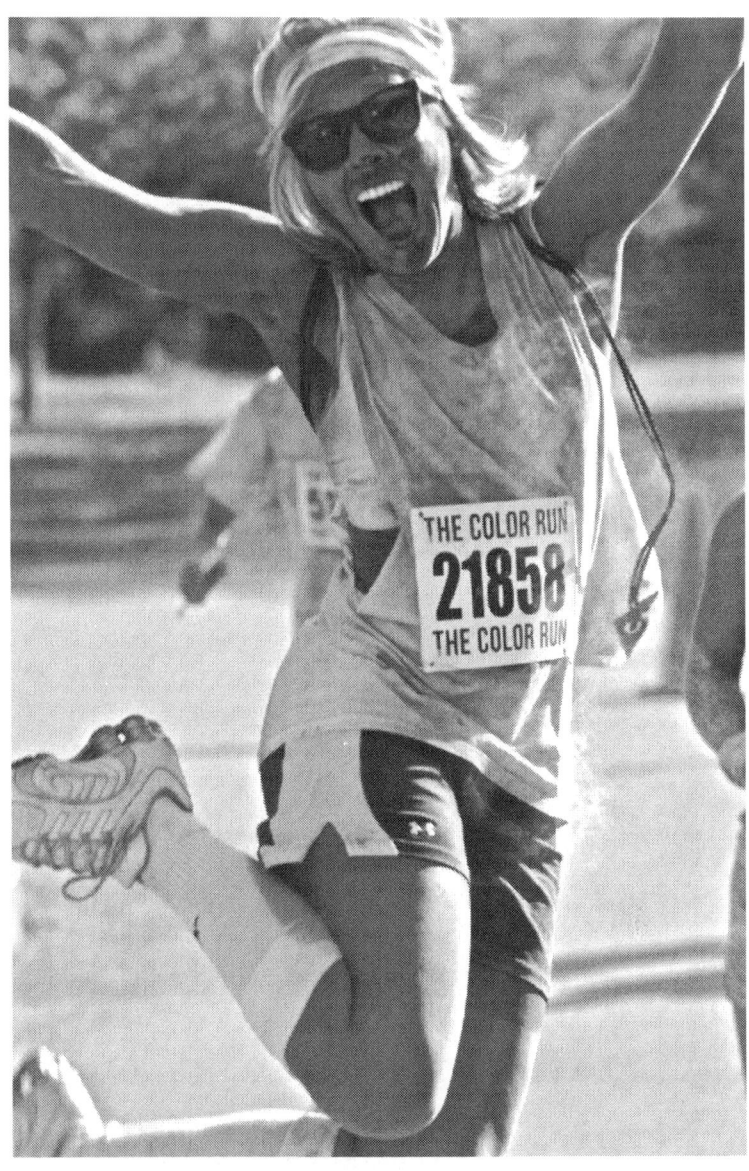

When choosing a race, keep it fun. Races don't have to be serious.

(The Pug Father - CC BY 2.0)

Equipment

Running is the most basic sport there is and yet there is tons of equipment available for it. After you finish Couch to 5K you might want to invest in some of the extras, but to get started you really just need the basics.

Shoes

You're going to be spending a lot of time in these shoes, so be sure that you like them. Buy a pair of running-specific shoes – not cross-trainers, walking shoes or other athletic shoes. When it comes to specific brands and models it's largely a matter of preference. Try your shoes on and don't be afraid to walk or even jog around the store before buying them. You might feel silly, but you'll soon learn that silly is the norm when it comes to runners. You don't need to spend a fortune on running shoes, but that being said if you're going to splurge in one area I recommend investing in good shoes.

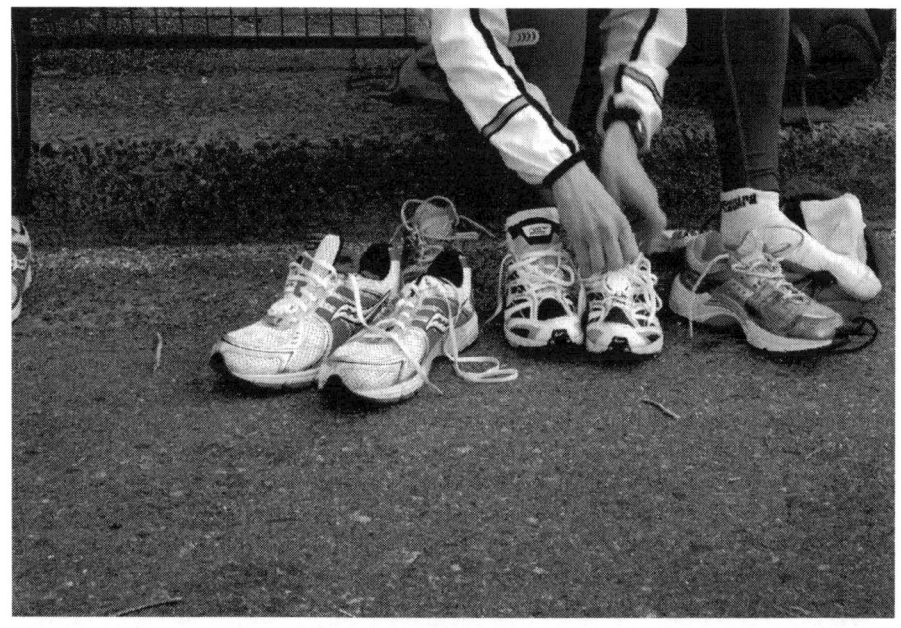

Select a pair of shoes that's right for you. (Kris Krug – CC BY-SA 2.0)

Clothing

If you're running in warm weather or indoors, then clothing is easy. A simple t-shirt and shorts is sufficient for most people. Some runners will tell you to stay away from cotton because it holds sweat close to the body, but for the purposes of Couch to 5K it's fine. If you're running in cold weather then clothing becomes more important. When it's cold you should dress in layers and wear synthetics that will wick sweat away from your skin.

One must-have for women – regardless of the weather – is a good sports bra. A sports bra will hold your breasts in place, making your run much more comfortable.

Gadgets

There are oodles of gadgets available for runners, from simple stopwatches to GPS tracking devices.

You will need a means of timing yourself. A stopwatch will do the trick but you don't necessarily need one if you're using an app or podcast that times you – in which case you'll need a smartphone, iPod or another mp3 player.

I recommend getting a stopwatch with a heart rate monitor. A heart rate monitor will track your heart rate over your run so you know just how hard you're pushing yourself. There are two basic types of heart rate monitors: ones that you touch to get an instant reading from and ones that give a continuous reading via a strap that you wear around your chest. For running you really need the latter type.

I now run with a GPS watch to track my distance and pace. It's a must-have for a serious marathon runner or anyone doing speed work, but it's not necessary for a novices. Consider it in the future, but for now it's not a necessity.

Apps and Podcasts

Theoretically you can do the Couch to 5K program with nothing more than a stopwatch to time yourself, but I don't recommend it. Using an app or a podcast that times your runs lets you concentrate on running instead of worrying about timing.

Active.com has an official app based on Josh Clark's original Couch to 5K program for both iOS and Android. Other apps exist, though they may vary from the original program.

Another option is to use a podcast – which is what I did. You can simply download a series of Couch to 5K podcasts that will tell you when to run or walk. I used Robert Ullrey's podcasts which are available for free on iTunes and c25K.com. By week 7, when you are just running without walk breaks, then you can do away with the podcast and simply use a stopwatch.

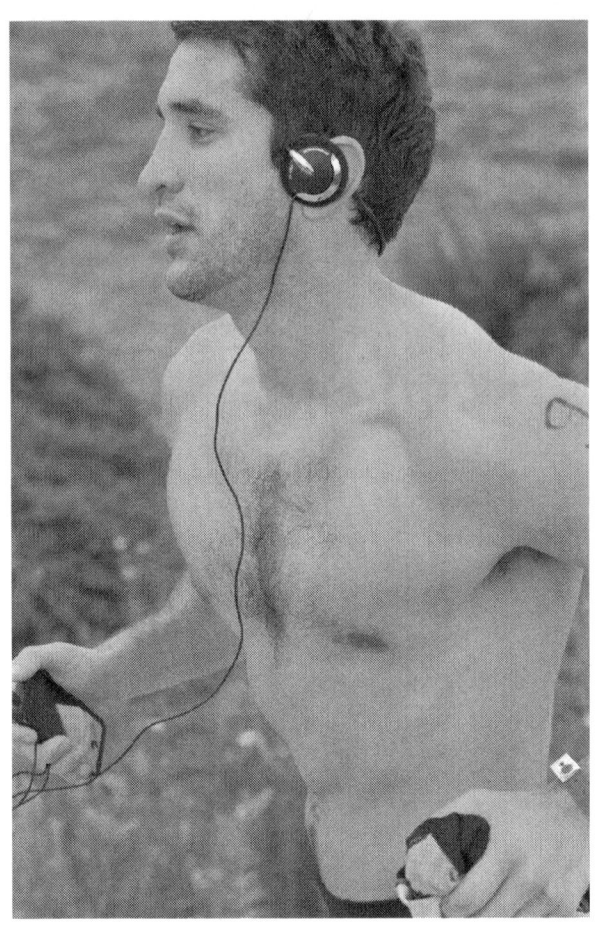

Listening to music can be a welcome distraction. (Chris Hunkelar –
CC BY 2.0)

Warm-up and Cool Down

Each Couch to 5K workout begins with a warm-up walk and ends with a cool down walk. If you're tempted to save time or energy by cutting out this portion of the workout, forget about it! The warm-up and cool down are essential components of the workout if you want to avoid getting hurt.

Warming up gets your heart rate up and loosens up your muscles. This prepares your muscles for action and will reduce your chances of injury. The recommended warm-up for Couch to 5K is simple; walk briskly for 5 minutes. That's it. After your 5-minute walk your muscles should be sufficiently warmed up.

After your workout there's a good chance that you'll be pretty tired. Even if you are exhausted, you can't just stop your workout cold. If you sit down or lay down at the end of your workout then your blood pressure and heart rate can drop quickly, leaving you light-headed. Use a 5-minute walk at the end of your workout to gradually reduce your heart rate.

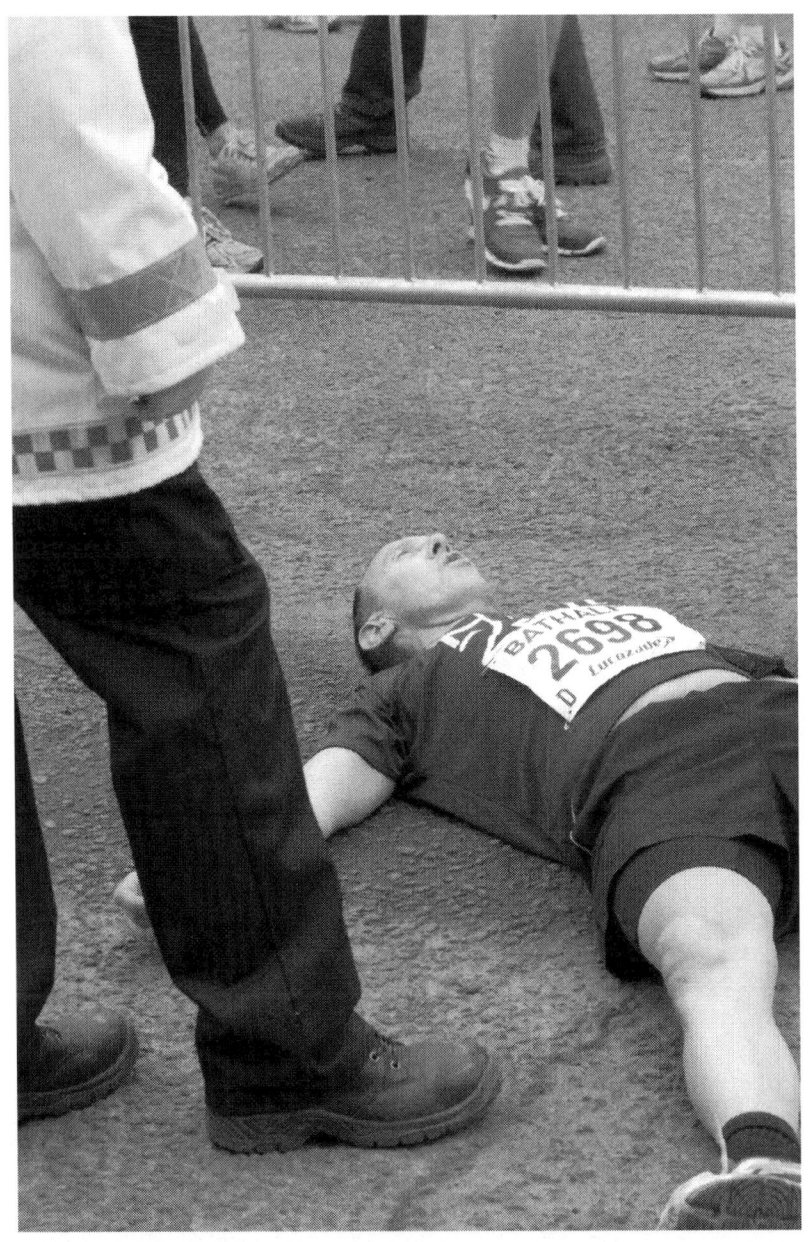

Don't rest immediately after running – no matter how tempting it may be. (Stephen Shellard – CC BY 2.0)

Stretches

After warming up you're not quite ready to start your run. To loosen up your muscles and avoid injury you should stretch before jumping into the real workout. It's important to do your stretches *after* the warm-up, not before it, because muscles stretch better when they are warm. You should also stretch after the cool down to minimize any aches and pains after running.

Running obviously works your leg muscles the most, so they are the focus of your stretches. Specifically, you should stretch your calves, hamstrings, quadriceps and groin.

You can use the same basic stretches after both the warm-up and cool down. Do each of the following stretches two or three times, holding each stretch for 15 to 30 seconds.

Calf Stretches

Position yourself 3 feet away from a wall with your feet shoulder's width apart (in a pinch another sturdy surface like a tree or a lamppost will do in place of a wall). Place your hands on the wall with your arms parallel to the floor. Lean your hips forward and bend your knees slightly while keeping your feet on the ground. You should feel your calves stretching as you do this.

Bend over from your position in the first stretch so your torso is parallel with the floor and your arms are braced against the wall. Move your feet back if necessary to keep your arms stretched out. Bring one foot forward with your knee bent slightly. Lift the toe of your front foot to stretch the calf. Switch the position of your feet and perform the stretch on the opposite calf.

Again from the same position, place your feet together and lift the toes of both of your feet. As you do so, rock back onto your heels and push against the wall.

Hamstring Stretch

Lie down on your back. Bend one knee with your foot on the ground. Raise the other leg straight up in the air. Grab the raised leg and pull on it as you push with it against your hands. Reverse the position of your legs and perform the stretch on the opposite leg.

Quadriceps Stretch

Stand on one foot, bracing yourself against a solid object if necessary. Raise the other foot back, up toward your butt and hold it with your opposite hand. Keep your body as upright as possible and push your pelvis forward to really work your quads. Repeat this stretch with the opposite leg.

Groin Stretch

Sit on the ground and place the soles of your feet together. Place your elbows on the inside of your knees and your hands on your ankles. Gently press your knees down with your elbows, stretching out the groin.

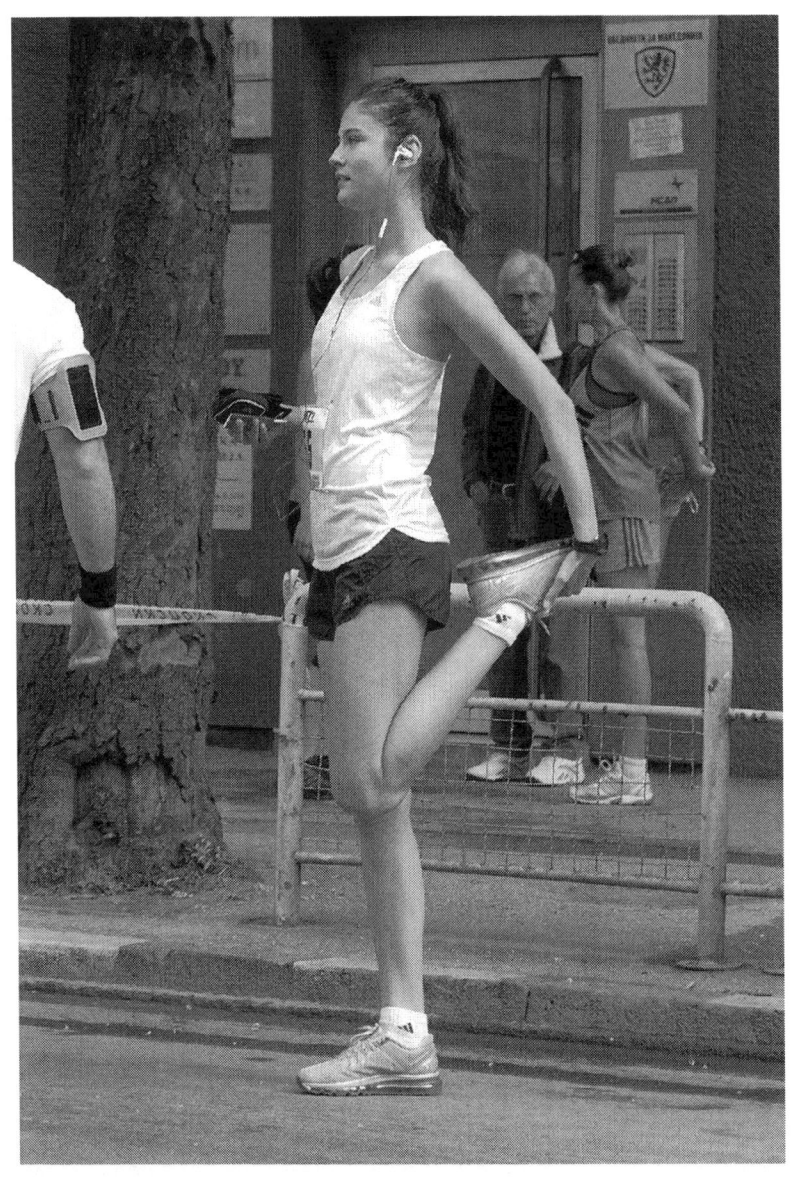

You can use two hands for quad stretches, if you prefer. (Marjan Lazarevski – CC BY-ND 2.0)

The Program

Couch to 5K is a nine week running program. Each week you will have three runs. You can schedule these runs as you please, but they should be spread out across the week so that you are never running two days in a row. This is important because your body needs rest. As you improve as a runner and build strength you may be able to run more than three times a week, but until then you need to protect your body from injury.

Couch to 5K uses a combination of running and walking in the early parts of the program, making it easier for you to get started. Each week the amount of running will increase relative to the amount of walking until you are running exclusively. Then the length of your runs will increase gradually until you're running a full 5 Km.

Each run takes approximately 30 minutes. This includes a 5-minute warm-up walk at the beginning of each workout and a 5-minute cool down at the end.

Week 1

- Alternate running for 60 seconds and walking for 90 seconds for 20 minutes total (excluding the warm-up and cool down)

The first week of the program really eases you into things. You will be doing more walking than running during this week. Even though there isn't much running here, this is one of the harder weeks for a lot of people. If you're out of shape then running at all may be a challenge. Just be sure to pace yourself. If you're having difficulty breathing, slow down and take your time.

Week 2

- Alternate running for 90 seconds and walking for 180 seconds for 20 minutes total (excluding the warm-up and cool down)

In week 2 the length of the runs increases, but so does the length of the walks. 90 seconds may seem like a long time to run, but just remember it's a jog, not a sprint. Maintain an easy pace through the running portion and use the walking portions to recover. Two minutes can also seem like a long time for a walk, but remember that you need this time to recover. Don't cut your walks short even if you feel like you can handle more running.

Week 3

Do the following twice:

- Jog 200 yards (200 metres) or 90 seconds
- Walk 200 yards (200 metres) or 90 seconds
- Jog 400 yards (400 metres) or 3 minutes
- Walk 400 yards (400 metres) or three minutes

Things change a bit in week 3 because you can either continue measuring your runs/walks by time or you can do it by distance. The choice is really a matter of preference. If you're using an app or other device that measures your distance than that may be the easiest choice, but if you're using a podcast or a stopwatch then time is the only way to go.

Week 4

- Jog 1/4 mile (400 metres) or 3 minutes
- Walk 1/8 mile (200 metres) or 90 seconds
- Jog 1/2 mile (800 metres) or 5 minutes
- Walk 1/4 mile (400 metres) or 2-1/2 minutes
- Jog 1/4 mile (400 metres) or 3 minutes
- Walk 1/8 mile (200 metres) or 90 seconds
- Jog 1/2 mile (800 metres) or 5 minutes

By week 4 you should be ready to start some 5-minute runs. This week has one of the more confusing sets of intervals, so it's one where using a podcast or an app is highly advisable.

Week 5

Week 5 is a little different because you actually have three different sets of intervals for the three runs.

First Run:

- Jog 1/2 mile (800 metres) or 5 minutes
- Walk 1/4 mile (400 metres) or 3 minutes
- Jog 1/2 mile (800 metres) or 5 minutes
- Walk 1/4 mile (400 metres) or 3 minutes
- Jog 1/2 mile (800 metres) or 5 minutes

Second Run:

- Jog 3/4 mile (1.2 Km) or 8 minutes
- Walk 1/2 mile (800 metres) or 5 minutes
- Jog 3/4 mile (1.2 Km) or 8 minutes

Third Run:

- Jog 2 miles (3.2 Km) or 20 minutes

The third run of the week is the most difficult for many people because it makes a pretty dramatic leap to a 2-mile or 20-minute run without any walk breaks. If you have trouble with stamina, don't be discouraged if you need to attempt this run more than once (see the section below on modifying the program).

Week 6

In week 6 you will also have three different sets of intervals.

First Run:

- Jog 1/2 mile (800 metres) or 5 minutes
- Walk 1/4 mile (400 metres) or 3 minutes
- Jog 3/4 mile (1.2 Km) or 8 minutes
- Walk 1/4 mile (400 metres) or 3 minutes

- Jog 1/2 mile (800 metres) or 5 minutes

Second Run:

- Jog 1 mile (1.6 Km) or 10 minutes
- Walk 1/4 mile (400 metres) or 3 minutes
- Jog 1 mile (1.6 Km) or 10 minutes

Third Run

- Run 2-1/4 miles (3.6 Km) or 22 minutes

Week 7

After week 6 you're through with walking (except for your warm-up and cool down). Week 7 simply picks up where week 6 finished. You'll run for 2.5 miles (4 Km) or 25 minutes.

Week 8

In week 8 you'll push yourself just a bit further. You will run for 2.75 miles (4.5 Km) or 28 minutes. By this point you should be almost ready to run a 5K.

Week 9

Week 9 marks the end of the program. At this point you should be able to run approximately 5 Km. According to the imperial version of the program you will actually run 3 miles, which at 4.83 Km is just shy of a full 5K. If you want you can plan to run a 5K race during this week, but you may want to attempt a few runs on your own before participating in a race.

Pacing Yourself

As you get in better shape it can be tempting to pick up the pace and run as fast as you can during Couch to 5K. Fight the urge to do this. Maintain a comfortable pace as you run. You shouldn't be completely out of breath. A good test, if you're running with a partner, is if you can maintain a conversation. If you're too out of breath to talk comfortably, then you're going too fast. Remember, the goal of the Couch to 5K program isn't to build speed, it's to build distance. When it comes to the walking portions it's alright to push yourself a little harder. If you need more of a challenge, walk at your maximum walking speed. Just don't let it turn into a run.

Modifying the Program

The Couch to 5K program is intended to last 9 weeks, but this is really just a guideline. Depending on your ability it may take you longer to complete the program. If at some point in the program you don't feel like you're ready to move on to the next week or the next run, that's alright. Just repeat the previous run or week until you feel ready to move on. If you can't finish a run don't worry either, just attempt it again for your next run or consider moving back to the previous week. Don't try to cram extra runs into the week if you're struggling though; limit yourself to three runs per week and simply extend the number of weeks in the program.

If your runs are going well you may be tempted to skip ahead in the program. People sometimes do this when they sign up for a 5K a month away and then realize they need to get in shape. I really have to advise against this. If you push yourself too hard you're going to risk injury. As Josh Clark says, "It's important to resist [skipping ahead], to give your body a chance to get used to all this new activity." So be patient and take your time with the program. Remember, 9 weeks really isn't very long and it will take a lot longer if you injure yourself.

Before You Quit

Like any workout regimen, Couch to 5K has dropouts. Don't be one. The program may get tough for you. You may get off track. But don't let these be reasons to quit altogether.

If the program gets too hard for you, just take a step back (as discussed in the section on modifying the program). Remember, you've already made progress and you will make more if you give yourself time. If you need to redo a week three times before moving on it's better than walking away.

If you fall off track, get back on track as fast as possible. The sooner you get back to running, the easier it will be. But if you wait too long you'll lose your cardiovascular fitness. You may be able to jump right back into the program, but if it's been a while you'll probably have to go back a few weeks. Pick a week that's comfortable for you and start from there. If it's still too hard, move back even further. In a worst case scenario you'll need to restart. You don't want to put yourself in a position where that happens, but if you find yourself there don't despair. I know Couch to 5K graduates who didn't make it on the first or even second try, but they're happy they came back.

Before you give up, think about the reasons that you started the program – and that you should have written down before starting.

Use this as your motivation to get through the program.

After Couch to 5K

After you finish the Couch to 5K program you'll be able to run 3 miles or 5 Km. What you do with this new found ability is up to you. But whatever you decide, be sure to do something. If you stop running at the end of the program then you will gradually lose your running ability.

You may simply want to continue casually running 5 Km a few times a week. If that's what you want to do then it's great! That's a fantastic way to get exercise and maintain your running abilities.

If you enjoy 5K races then you might want to stick with the distance and work on your speed. I won't go into the details of speed training, but there are a lot of ways to improve your times. Interval training, hill training and distance runs can all be used as part of a 5K training program. You'll also want to work on the technical side of running, perfecting your stride length and rate (don't worry about this during Couch to 5K though).

Couch to 5K gets you in the habit of pushing your distance limit, so when the program ends you may want to keep increasing your distances. There are countless training programs for building up to a 10K, half marathon or even a full marathon (though the latter takes considerably more training).

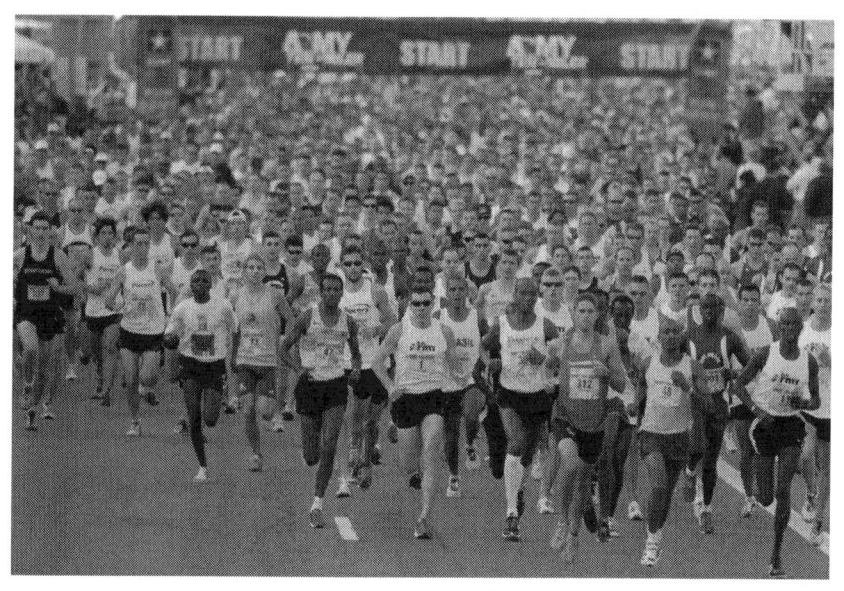

Your options are limitless after finishing Couch to 5K. (U.S. Army MWR – CC BY 2.0)

31713325R00035

Made in the USA
Middletown, DE
09 May 2016